no
SWEAT

An Introduction To Spread-Workouts
And The 3-6-10 Health And Body Shaper.

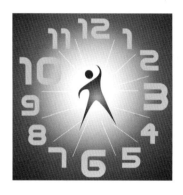

Shedding Light on a More Convenient
Way to Exercise

no SWEAT

*An Introduction To Spread-Workouts
And The 3-6-10 Health And Body Shaper.*

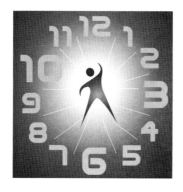

*Shedding Light on a More Convenient
Way to Exercise*

**RYAN PENNY and SEAN PENNY
THE WELLNESS BROTHERS**

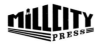

Mill City Press, Inc.
212 3rd Avenue North, Suite 290
Minneapolis, MN 55401
612.455.2294
www.millcitypublishing.com

ISBN-13: 978-1-62652-009-7
LCCN: 2013901541

Cover Design by Mary Ross
Typeset by James Arneson

Printed in the United States of America

Images 1, 13, 16: Copyright 2004, Progressive Sporting Systems, reprinted with permission

Images 2, 3, 4, 5, 6, 7, 9, 10, 12, 14, 15: Copyright 2011, Physigraphe, reprinted with permission

The information in this book is not intended to be and does not constitute medical advice. As with all programs, techniques, and materials related to health, exercise, fitness, and weight loss, the authors recommend that you use proper discretion in conjunction with your physician or other health care professional in using the information presented. The author and publisher expressly disclaim responsibility for any adverse effects that may result from the use or application of the information contained in this book.

Dedicated to Donna, Hannah, and Kelsey, the ones who inspire us to push our Spread-Workouts that little bit harder.

CONTENTS

Exercise has never been more convenient

FOREWORD

IT'S NO SECRET that people are becoming increasingly sedentary as they enjoy the ease and convenience of technology. The irony is that the lack of physical activity robs millions of people of true ease and comfort by compounding obesity and other chronic diseases.

The good news is that this book can make a difference.

If you had to ask me whether it contains all you need to know about fitness and exercise, I would answer no. But that's clearly not the intention. *NO SWEAT* was written with one goal in mind: *to help people get out of the trap of a sedentary lifestyle in the most convenient way possible.*

In an industry where there is no shortage of material, this book's shear simplicity and ease of application sets it apart. True to form, the Wellness Brothers have identified the heart of the problem and offered us a genuine and doable solution.

No more excuses.

Let's exercise.

Dr. Manoj Kumar, M.D.
Physical & Rehabilitation Medicine

INTRODUCTION

How less became more

RYAN AND I have always been active. Since we were children, we've spent countless hours in the swimming pool, on the soccer field, playing golf, and running around the squash court. For us, competitive sports have been a way of life.

But, like most people, when we started to work, things slowed down. The days became increasingly demanding, and the time we had for all our games seemed to evaporate. Like virtually every person who came to our practice, we were finding it difficult to fit our exercise into the busyness of life.

In 2006, Ryan and his wife, Bronwyn, had Donna, the first of their three beautiful girls. Not too long after that it was clear to me that a growing family made regular exercise even more of a challenge. When Hannah, their second child, was born, Ryan's sport came to almost a complete stop. While I continued playing a reasonable amount of squash and soccer, he did little more than play a bit golf and occasionally meet me on the squash court.

Yet, despite his massive drop off in activity, I wasn't the only one who noticed that Ryan seemed to maintain a good level of fitness. Most of the people who knew him well were inclined to say that he'd been blessed with good genes. They assumed that he was just one of those guys who was naturally fit. I must say, I thought the same until one day I made an interesting discovery.

Ryan had actually been exercising almost daily for years. It wasn't as if he was trying to hide it; it was just that he had incorporated physical activity into his day in a way that few people ever saw. In fact, only Bronwyn and the girls really knew that he was in the habit of squeezing exercise in between other things.

While he ran his morning bathwater, he would work out with a piece of surgical tubing. He would do push-ups and squats while bathing the kids and waiting for his smoothie to mix in the blender. When he would get home from work, he would do two or three minutes of tuck-jumps, sprints on the spot, and bicycle-crunches. He felt this was a great way to clear his head after a hectic day and separate his time at work and his time at home. As it turns out, Ryan's shape and fitness, which seemed unusual for somebody who was apparently doing so little, was not that extraordinary after all. The secret was not hidden in his DNA but, rather, wrapped up in his *convenient approach* to staying in shape.

Ryan's way of making movement fit into his day rather than shuffling his day to fit in with his movement also went a step further. After reading about a study that showed how overweight people spent significantly more time sitting than those considered "normal" weight, and in an attempt to show his weight-loss patients that it was possible to increase their physical activity without going to the gym, he remodelled his consulting room. He exchanged the chairs for large, blue physio balls. He brought in a treadmill so that consultations could be done while his patients walked. Some people thought he took it too far when he got rid of all the waiting room chairs, but Ryan was convinced that every bit of movement counted, and he wanted people to benefit whenever and wherever they could.

Over the past three years I've been using the in-between approach to exercise, too. I can honestly say that my experience has been great, which is one of the main reasons I want to share our 3-6-10 approach with you; more about that at the end of chapter 2, though. All you need to know at this point is that NO SWEAT is a summary of what Ryan and I now do all the time.

As you continue reading, so you'll discover all you need to know to enjoy the same benefits that we have. To ensure you do, I'd like you to approach this book with the same mindset that you'd have building a puzzle. In other words, I want you to be prepared to piece everything together to get the whole Spread-Workout picture. That means being willing to read the whole book, an overview of which looks like this.

In the opening chapter, Ryan's going to show you "the cover of the box" to reveal the bigger picture. In chapters 2 through 7 he will "open the box" to start sorting through the pieces and putting them together. Let me assure you that, even though you might think it at times, there aren't any pieces missing. Everything you need is here, and by the time Ryan is done with the seventh chapter you will have just about finished piecing it together. In chapter 8, I will pick things up again and make sure that your *NO-SWEAT* picture is complete. But, before I hand this over to Ryan, there are three things that I want to clarify.

The first is that a good diet is an essential part of a lifestyle aimed at better health, shape, and function. Ryan and I firmly believe this. *NO SWEAT*, however, is about movement and not food. Apart from what I touch on briefly in the final chapter, you won't read anything about what to eat. Again, that's not because we don't think it's important, it's just that this book is not our platform for that discussion.

The next thing might sound obvious, but it's important to explain what we mean by a "rep" and a "set" in the context of the book. A rep is a single, complete movement of *any* exercise. A set is the period of time, no matter how long or short, in which reps are accumulated.

The third thing is that it's our intention for this book to be practical. That's why at regular intervals you will be prompted to get up and exercise. Please don't neglect this aspect of the book. As you will see, every time you move your body, you move yourself toward being a healthier, more functional, and better shaped individual.

Okay, that's it from me for now. It's time for Ryan to expand on what I've said and show you how you can enjoy the benefits of the 3-6-10 Spread-Workouts, an anytime, anywhere, equipment-free form of exercise training.

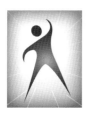

CHAPTER 1

Spread-Workouts

A convenient solution for everybody

EXERCISE IS THE most beneficial thing for your health. It also produces a firm and shapely body. Over and above the well-known advantages of weight loss, lower cholesterol, and better blood sugar control, exercise adds spice to life by improving things like:

- Energy levels
- Concentration
- Strength
- Speed
- Agility
- Sexual function
- Sleep

Perhaps the best thing about regular exercise is that the rewards extend to everybody. Regardless of your age, gender, or state of health, you stand to profit from doing more physical activity. But isn't it this *doing* part that's just the problem? After all, there are so many obstacles.

Sean and I constantly hear things like, "I have no time," "It's too difficult," "I don't know what to do," "Gyms are too expensive," and "I just don't like to get sweaty." These kinds of excuses keep millions of people from better health, shapelier bodies, and other benefits like the ones I mentioned. In fact, recent research[1] suggests that physical inactivity—defined as failure to do fifteen to thirty minutes of brisk walking a day—increases the risk of cancer, heart disease, stroke, and diabetes by twenty to thirty percent. What may come as a real surprise is that inactivity is as dangerous as smoking.

In 2008, tobacco and sedentary behavior killed a combined total of more than ten million people.[2] Each habit accounted for over five million deaths, which, I think, are best described as protracted suicides. The reality is that people today are quite literally sitting themselves to death.

But, it doesn't have to be this way. Being more physically active is well within the reach of everybody. All of the time, effort, know-how, cost, and preference hurdles can be overcome with the 3-6-10 Spread-Workout strategy that I'm about to unpack for you.

Breaking it up

Imagine that you and three friends are going on a road trip. You've all agreed on where to go, have planned the route, and are excited to be leaving the next day. Early the following morning you arrive at the friend's house whose car you're all travelling in, and there, standing behind the open trunk of the vehicle, the three of them are waiting with their luggage. Each has a single, large suitcase, similar to yours, and what's obvious is that there's not enough space for everybody's stuff. Being last to arrive, it seems you will be the one who has to stay behind.

Not wanting to miss out, you do some quick thinking to find a solution. "What if I pack all my stuff into smaller bags?" you say to your friends. "The ones that don't fit in the trunk can go under the seats, at our feet, and behind our heads in the back." Your friends, who would love for you to join them, agree to your plan, and a short while later, after some skilful baggage Tetris, everything is in and you're all on your way.

Now, if you've ever packed a car, or anything else for that matter, you know that, depending on the space available, too many large items make for a headache. When space is limited, smaller things can be squeezed in where bigger things can't. The same is true for exercise.

If you don't have the time for thirty-, forty-, or sixty-minute workouts in the gym, that doesn't mean exercise needs to be left out altogether. Instead, you can break it up, re-package it, and spread it out in a way that fits into your day. Ten quick push-ups before your shower, fifteen shallow squats before you get in the car, or five speedy stick-ups before you sit down at your desk are examples of exercise being split up and slotted in.

One of the nice things is it doesn't matter whether you are fit or unfit to begin with; this novel approach to moving away from the risks of being sedentary is viable for everybody. It's an ideal way for non-exercisers to get started and for people who are used to doing longer, single sessions to supplement their workouts. In the end, it doesn't matter whether you are in peak physical condition or totally out of shape—the Spread-Workout Solution can work for you.

Mentally and physically effective

The place that Spread-Workouts have their initial impact is on the mind. They help overcome limiting beliefs about exercise. You see, if you, like many people, are trapped into believing that only long and strenuous workouts are good for your health and shape, you will not be inclined to consider doing anything short. The idea of five reps before you leave the office or ten in the kitchen before you prepare dinner would make no sense; it would seem like a wasted effort and you wouldn't do it.

But, that all changes when you appreciate how beneficial Spread-Workouts can actually be. Confidence in the effectiveness of short-bout exercise accumulation frees you up. It opens your eyes to more movement opportunities than you would otherwise see when blinded by an all-or-nothing exercise mentality. The reality is that every bit of physical activity, done safely of course, is good for you. This is something you need to believe, which is why I want you to carefully consider what comes next.

More is great, but a little is good enough

Research has shown that the largest health gain from exercise is for inactive people. When they do as little as fifteen minutes a day they stand to enjoy the greatest proportional benefit.[3]

That's not to say that more isn't better; it just means that the little bit done at the beginning is where things help the most.

Yet, proof that a small amount is beneficial doesn't necessarily say anything about exercise *accumulation*, which is what Spread-Workouts are all about. That's why the next bit of evidence is so important.

In a study done on overweight women, it was shown that three ten-minute bouts of exercise done through the day enhanced weight loss and produced similar changes in cardio-respiratory fitness to those who had exercised in the more traditional, long-bout way. What's more, the short bouts also improved exercise adherence, suggesting that they may be preferred when prescribing exercise to obese adults.[4] As far as Sean and I can tell, the improvement in compliance is not unique to obese women. The convenience of spreading things out seems to appeal to many different people who want to do more exercise more consistently.

Rationale for the 3-6-10 Spread-Workouts

There is good evidence to support the health and shape benefits of accumulating short bouts of exercise throughout the day. In general, however, the research I'm referring to has typically involved cardio exercise, like walking, and for durations of ten minutes. This is different from what Sean and I are recommending in our Spread-Workouts. Instead of ten-minute sessions, much *shorter* stints are performed, and in place of cardio exercises, *bodyweight* exercises are used.

To decide whether the variance detracts from the value of the 3-6-10 approach, I think it's helpful to answer two questions:

1. *Are the individual bouts long enough to be of benefit?*
2. *Are bodyweight exercises comparable with the cardio ones in the research done on the overweight women?*

I will begin with the first one.

In 2010, I met Professor John Jakicic. The man is a giant in the field of exercise research and is known for his studies in the areas of the varying doses of exercise on long-term weight control, the use of intermittent exercise to promote the adoption and maintenance of physical activity in overweight adults, and the use of behavioral strategies to improve long-term weight loss outcomes.

In what were, ironically, only a few brief chats spread over three days, I specifically asked him how the decision was made about the duration of the exercises done in the study I cited on the overweight women. I wanted to know if he considered the ten-minute mark some kind of threshold at which physical activity becomes beneficial. His replies were enlightening.

Professor Jakicic explained that the ten-minute recommendation primarily factored in two things. The first was a *physical consideration* based on the fact that it takes around five minutes of physical activity for the body to properly ready itself for more intense cardiovascular exercise. A ten-minute session was a logical conclusion, as it made room for a warm-up and left time for additional activity. The second reason was based on how people were likely to *perceive* a short-bout approach. The thinking was that, for most people, ten minutes would seem both convenient and meaningful enough to do and therefore motivate compliance. When the physical and mental pieces were put together, ten minutes was the *magic number* for the research.

By the end of our discussions, Professor Jakicic and I agreed that, from the perspective of benefit, the magic number was not so magic after all. The nine minutes and fifty-nine seconds leading up to it are not a necessary evil to breaking through some kind of benefit barrier. Instead, all the time spent getting to the ten-minute mark is also valuable. When you look at it in this way, it's hard not to conclude that, when done safely, physical activity is good for you from the moment you start moving.

More recently, scientists have begun to recognize that the time we spend doing *sedentary things*, like sitting, can have a direct negative impact on health. A growing body of research suggests that even people who exercise regularly but spend most of their days at a desk, on the couch, or in the car are at greater risk of disease than active people who walk around and move a lot through the day. What is becoming clear is that single-session workouts are not enough for optimal health. That's not to say they aren't good—they are—but they need to be supported by regular interruptions in time spent in low-energy states of minimal muscle activity.

Now, think about it. If the goal is to accumulate ten, fifteen, or maybe twenty minutes of exercise for the day in bouts lasting only a few seconds to a few minutes, how many times will you need get up and move? That's right, probably between four and twenty times. Well, guess what that does to long periods of sitting? It fragments it brilliantly, adding support to the value of very short bouts of exercise, which we have already concluded are beneficial from the moment the movement begins.

In summary, the combination of physical exercise accumulated throughout the day and the regular disruptions in sitting facilitated by very short-bout Spread-Workouts can be highly effective at improving health, reducing the risk of multiple diseases, and enhancing body shape.

With this in mind, let's move on to the second question: Are the bodyweight exercises used in the 3-6-10 approach as effective as the cardio ones done in the research?

The short answer is no.

That's because the bodyweight exercises are even *more* effective.

You see, bodyweight exercises have a three-dimensional impact. Not only do they have a good *cardio effect* when they are done for more than a minute and a half, but they also build greater strength and improve co-ordination. The bodyweight exercises included in the 3-6-10 approach have been selected because, together, they work just about the whole body. This makes for more intense workouts, superior fat burn, and firmer muscles.

All in all, compound bodyweight exercises provide a bigger bang for your buck. They can make you fitter, stronger, and better balanced, allowing you to enjoy greater health, better shape, and a lower risk of physical injury in the course of daily life.

Piecing it together before moving on

I'm sure that you will agree that in light of what I've been telling you, the research supporting the benefit of short-bout exercise accumulation can be stretched to support the 3-6-10 approach's use of even shorter bouts of bodyweight exercises.

Beyond the research, however, it has been Sean's and my experience that our approach offers a *convenient* way of moving more and moving more often. It's effective and flexible, making it suitable for just about anybody. Personalizing it to suit you is straightforward, and in the coming chapters you will see just how to do that.

As you go about deciding on the 3-6-10 plan that best suits you, be sure to focus on safety. This is something I will repeatedly remind you of. If you choose to begin doing the Spread-Workouts before you get to the final chapter in which Sean summarizes how best to do them, just be sure to begin as slowly as you need to. When you get the feel of how it all works, and as you get stronger and fitter, you can aim to do more and more. This way you will enjoy the greatest benefits.

Now, before you move on to chapter 2 where I will show you how to go about finding the right fit for you, I want you to stand up, stretch your hands above your head, and walk at least ten steps. If you feel up to it, add ten jumping-jacks after the walk; that's exactly what I'm about to do.

"Lack of activity destroys the good condition of every human being while movement and methodical exercise save and preserve it." **– Plato**

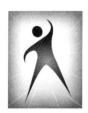

CHAPTER 2

The Right Fit

It's best when it suits you

PICTURE YOURSELF walking into a shoe store and looking for a new pair of shoes to workout in. As you scout around, you are bombarded by brands and adverts of all different colors, shapes, and sizes. Things are so bright and busy that it's difficult to know where to begin. Fortunately, the store assistant recognizes your deer-in-headlights look and heads over to lend a hand.

"Hi, my name's Frank. Can I help you?"

"Yes, please. I'm looking for a pair of shoes I can run in and use in the gym. I don't plan on doing too much distance, and I want something comfortable."

Frank nods. "I think we've got just what you need."

He leads you over to a separate display area and picks up what looks more like a glove for your foot than a shoe. Frank smiles at your obvious doubt and assures you that he's not having you on. "They are quite new," he says, "but so many people who have bought them rave about how good they are.

You can run in them, use them in the gym, and even just wear them around the house. Let me get you a pair to see how they fit. What's your size?" You tell him, and off he goes to the storeroom.

When he gets back, he's carrying three boxes. "I've got three different sizes for you to try on. There isn't really a direct conversion from your regular shoe size, and because people's feet can be so different, it's always best for you to put on a few pairs to see what suits you. The idea is for your heel to fit comfortably and for your longest toe to lightly touch the end of the pocket it's in."

You take a box, flip off the lid, and slip on the first pair. They look rather strange, like gorilla's feet, but after walking up and down a few times you actually start liking the idea of working out in them.

"How do they feel?" Frank asks.

"Different, but actually pretty good; it's almost as if I'm not wearing shoes at all."

"That sounds about right. You sure they aren't too loose? These shoes should be a snug fit; maybe even a little tight when they're new because they will stretch after you have worn them a few times."

"I wouldn't say they're snug. They're comfortable right now, but if you say they're likely to stretch, then let me try on another pair."

You sit down, make the change to the smaller size, then walk around again.

"I'm not sure, Frank. How tight is too tight?"

"If your toes are scrunched then that's no good. If your foot feels as if it's been squeezed gently, that should be fine. Do you think you could go for a run in them without having sore toes when you're done?"

"I think so. If they do stretch the way you say, then I imagine these are the ones."

"Fantastic," Frank says. "I suggest you take them home and wear them around the house for a few days. If you feel they aren't right, you can always bring them back and we can find another pair."

Specially for you

At some point in our lives, we've probably all worn shoes that weren't the right size for us. Either they were too big and tended to slip off, or they were too small, which made walking a painful experience. I remember playing squash a couple times in a pair too small for me. Instead of taking the time to try both shoes on when I bought them, I only put on the left one. It felt fine there in the shop, but I forgot that my left foot is slightly smaller than my right. The result was a bruising battle between my right big toe and the front of the shoe. In the end, the shoe won.

When things aren't the right fit, whether they're shoes, underpants, or airplane seats, things can get nasty. The same is true for exercise. Blisters, bruises, and even broken bones can result from doing workouts that are a poor match for you, even though they're perfect for somebody else. That's why it's important to find the right 3-6-10 fit for you.

To do that, there are a few things to consider. These include the actual 3-6-10 *exercises*; your current level of *fitness* (conditioning); your daily *routine*; and your personal *preferences*. To begin with let's talk about the exercises.

The 3-6-10 exercises

The first step to the right fit is choosing the exercises best for you. Unlike the shoe store where you met Frank, there aren't a whole lot of confusing options with the 3-6-10 plan. In fact, there are only five basic exercises that make up the whole program. That's not to say that other exercises are no good or that you can't include different ones in your Spread-Workouts; it's just that these are ideal to start out with. Here they are:

1. Push-ups
2. Squats
3. Cross-leg crunches
4. Mantis extensions
5. Wall stick-ups

Together these five exercises work the upper body, lower body, and core. Each exercise has progressions of difficulty, which means that you will easily find a variation to suit you. The push-ups, for example, can be done against a wall if you are an absolute beginner, from your knees when you are a little stronger, or like Spiderman when you are a lot stronger.

In the coming chapters, I will describe and illustrate each one of the exercises along with their variations and progressions.

As you read through them, I want you to mark off those that you think will best suit you to start out with. The progressions that might be too difficult for your current level of fitness should become targets for the future. In the end, progress in your health and shape will always be the result of progress in the intensity of the exercises and the number of reps you do.

The three fitness levels

If you are like most people, you have at least some idea of how fit and strong you are. You'll know whether you could do ten push-ups or a hundred, or whether you could run around the dining room table without stopping, or around the whole neighbourhood. As such, you can, in all probability, categorize yourself as being either *fit, average*, or *unfit*. Technically, that's enough to help you make many of your Spread-Workout decisions.

Rather than have you guess, though, we've included a *fitness estimation test* to help you classify yourself in 3-6-10 terms, namely *beginner*, *intermediate*, or *super-fit*. Knowing where you fit in will make your coming decisions easier and more appropriate.

The test itself only takes five minutes. So, as soon as you're done reading the instructions that follow, get up and do it. If, however, after taking a look at the test you feel that you won't be able to do either of the exercises, then *skip the test.* Simply take the five minutes that you would have spent doing the test to walk around. When you are done, turn to the heading

"Interpreting your results" on the next page and continue from there as a *beginner*.

The fitness estimation test

To complete your three-part fitness test, you need a pen and something to time yourself with. As long as you can see the start of each new minute, anything from a clock with a second hand to a stopwatch will do.

The test starts off with a three-minute warm-up. Immediately after that you will do as many push-ups as you can for one minute. Men do regular push-ups and women do knee push-ups. Following the push-ups, you will do as many shallow-squats as you can for another minute. If you are unsure of how to do either of the exercises and would like descriptions of them you can skip over to chapter 3 where you will find the regular push-ups on page 22, the knee push-ups on page 27, and the shallow squats on page 33. When you are satisfied that you know what to do, then come back to this point and begin the test.

In the space provided in the instructions, write down the number of push-ups and squats that you did. From there you can follow the guidelines for interpreting your results.

Are you ready?

Great, you can get started.

1. Warm-up

Begin with three minutes of alternate walking and jogging in place (on the spot). Switch every thirty seconds. Lift your knees higher and higher, swinging your arms more and more as the time passes. When three minutes are up, move quickly to the next exercise.

2. Push-ups

Do as many push-ups as you can in sixty seconds. Remember to do regular push-ups if you are male or knee push-ups if you are female.

My push-ups: _____

3. Shallow Squats

Immediately after completing the push-ups, do as many shallow squats as you can in sixty seconds.

My squats: _____

Interpreting your results

To determine your current 3-6-10 fitness level, you need to correlate your scores with the ones in the tables that follow. If both your upper and lower body test scores fit into the same category, then that's the appropriate level for you to get started with. If, however, your scores fall into two different categories, say, *intermediate* for push-ups and *beginner* for squats, then choose the lower of the two when you begin your 3-6-10 Spread-Workouts. For the example I just gave, that would be *beginner*.

As with choosing smaller shoes that are likely to stretch, opting for the lower level to begin with is always the better option because it reduces your injury risk and allows for a steady gain in fitness. Both are important for a good application of the system. With that in mind, go ahead and settle on your 3-6-10 fitness level.

Male fitness levels

Fitness Level	Regular Push-ups	Shallow Squats
Super-fit	> 50	> 50
Intermediate	> 25	> 25
Beginner	< 25	< 25

Female fitness levels

Fitness Level	Knee Push-ups	Shallow Squats
Super-fit	> 40	> 40
Intermediate	> 20	> 20
Beginner	< 20	< 20

Estimations are not absolutes

Something I want to make clear is that your 3-6-10 fitness level is *not* an absolute; it's a guide. Similar to when you buy shoes, the size you *commonly* wear is what's used to help the store assistant narrow things down. Rather than have someone, like Frank, bring out ten different sizes to try on, your usual size is the estimate that makes the selection process easier. Even so, it's still better to try on each pair to make sure that the ones you end up paying for are those that fit the best.

In the next two chapters I will describe and illustrate each of the 3-6-10 exercises. I will also include a recommendation with regards the suitability of each exercise for the different fitness levels. These are generalizations, so please don't assume that they're automatically right for you. You may well be able to include exercises recommended for higher fitness levels. That's fine. Just be careful. Also, if you are at intermediate or super-fit level, feel free to do any of the easier progressions. Pick and choose the way you would your shoes. If you are not entirely satisfied with the fit, you can always exchange them for others. That's something the 3-6-10 store encourages you to do.

Your daily routine and personal preferences

Not everybody finds the time to go looking for sports shoes. Neither is everybody fond of shoes that look like gorilla's feet. I say this to highlight the importance of factoring in your *daily routine* and *personal preferences* as you find a suitable 3-6-10 fit for you.

One of the nice things about the 3-6-10 approach is that it is extremely flexible. As you continue reading, you will see how easy it is to structure a Spread-Workout program that will fit in with who you are and what you do. Everything from here on is intended to show you how to personalize your anytime, anywhere, equipment-free exercise plan. In the end, it's ultimately up to you how you decide to use the information, but, in saying that, let me encourage you to aim for the 3-6-10 goal which, by the way, is where the program got its name:

- At least 3 sets a day
- 6 days a week
- Done in 10-week cycles

By the time you finish chapter 8, you will know exactly how to do this. In fact, I am confident that, no matter how busy you might be or what you like and don't like, this goal is within your reach. When you do achieve the 3-6-10 goal, you will enjoy its many health and body-shaping bonuses, which is why it's definitely something worth aiming for.

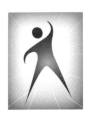

CHAPTER 3

Push-ups and Squats

Pillars of good health and better shape

BRICK AND MORTAR are to construction what push-ups and squats are to the 3-6-10. These two solid exercises are perfect for an equipment-free approach to Spread-Workouts.

In all probability you are already familiar with both of them. However, I suggest that you still read the whole chapter. Beyond what might be pure revision for you, there may be a few things that you'll pick up from the exercise descriptions, variations, and special tips that will improve your technique or add another dimension to the exercises.

Let's take it from the top.

1. Push-ups

The push-up is an outstanding upper body exercise that mainly works the chest, shoulders, and arms. When done properly—by holding the ankles, hips, and shoulders in a straight line—it also works the mid-section (core), buttocks, and thighs.

There are many progressions that can make a push-up easier or more difficult. These variations can also isolate specific muscles or recruit others, making the push-up a genuine multipurpose exercise. What follows is a description of how to do the movement properly.

1.1 Regular push-ups

Suitability: Beginner, intermediate, super-fit.
Begin by supporting your weight on your hands and toes, maintaining a straight body from your shoulders to your ankles.

Bend your elbows until your chest is just above the floor, and then push your weight back up until you have fully extended your arms.

Breathe in as you lower your body, and breathe out as you push up.

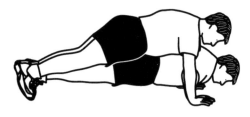

Useful tips for regular push-ups:

Tightening your buttocks and bracing your abs will help you maintain a straight body throughout the movement.

General push-up variations:

Where you place your hands and the *speed* at which you do your push-ups can alter the difficulty and effect of the exercise. Different hand positions and the timing of each rep are variations that can be applied to all the push-up progressions. These variations are also suitable for all three fitness levels.

Hand placements for push-up variations:

There are four different hand positions to use for any of the push-ups: close grip, medium stance, wide stance, and out of line.

1. Hands placed close together (close grip).

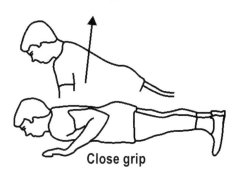

Close grip

The closer your hands are together, the closer you should keep your elbows to your sides through the movement. This will target the back of your arms (triceps) and your mid-chest.

2. Hands placed just beyond shoulder width (medium stance).

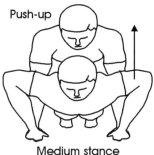

Push-up

Medium stance

As you place your hands farther apart, your elbows can move farther away from your body to work the outer part of chest more specifically.

- Hands placed wide apart (wide stance).

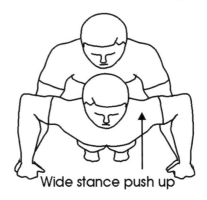

Wide stance push up

- Hands placed one in front of the other (out of line).

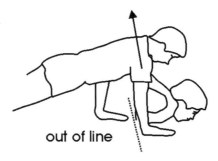

out of line

When opting for the staggered hand placement, make sure that your hands are about shoulder-width apart. Keep the elbow of the arm with the hand placed farther back tucked against your body through the movement. Let the elbow of the other arm move farther away from your body, the way it would when doing wide stance push-ups.

Remember to alternate so that you get an even number of reps with each hand in the front and back position. This is important for maintaining balance in muscle strength and development.

Timing for push-up variation:

There are obviously many different speeds at which the full push-up can be done. Here are the 3-6-10 recommendations:

- Fast: One second down, one second up.
- Medium: Two seconds down, one second up.
- Slow: Four seconds down, two seconds up.

Useful tips for timing:

The slower you lower your body and the faster you raise it up, the more intense the exercise. Another option for intensifying the movement is to hold the position at the bottom for an extra few seconds.

Timing can also be useful in completing a set. If you feel too tired to finish the one you are busy with, rather than stopping, it's a good idea to hold your position at the top, with your elbows "locked" for a few seconds, until you are ready to continue. This is another way to intensify your workouts.

Specific variations for push-ups:

There are four push-up progressions to choose from. Two of them are easier than the regular push-up and suited to beginners and intermediates. The other two are more difficult and best for the super-fit:

Easier push-ups:

- Wall push-ups
- Knee push-ups

More difficult push-ups:

- Spiderman push-ups
- Jump push-ups

1.2 Wall push-ups

Suitability: Beginner, intermediate.

These push-ups are the easiest of the lot and ideal for the overweight or anybody who has never done regular push-ups before.

Begin by standing about a foot and a half (or a little more as in the illustration) away from a solid wall. Place your hands on the wall just below shoulder level. Control your movement toward the wall with your arms until your nose just about touches the wall. Then push back to the starting position, keeping your elbows tight to your sides.

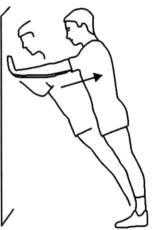

Useful tips for wall push-ups:

The same hand placement and timing variations for the regular push-ups can be applied to these. When you can do more than twenty wall push-ups without stopping, then you are ready to progress to the next level: the knee push-ups.

1.3 Knee push-ups

Suitability: Beginner, intermediate.
Begin by supporting your weight on your hands and knees in a kind of "all-fours" position with your ankles crossed. Bend your elbows, keeping them close to your sides until your chest is just above the floor. Push your weight up until you have fully extended your arms and are back in the starting position.

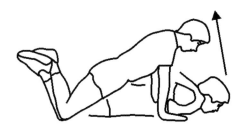

Useful tips for knee push-ups:

These knee push-ups are great for continuity. When fatigue hits while doing the more difficult push-ups, rather than stopping short of completing your set, you can keep going by dropping to your knees. This is a great way of doing that little bit extra, which can lead to better results.

1.4 Spiderman push-ups

Suitability: Intermediate, super-fit.
Spiderman push-ups are very demanding. They are best done when you want to add resistance and get your core more involved.

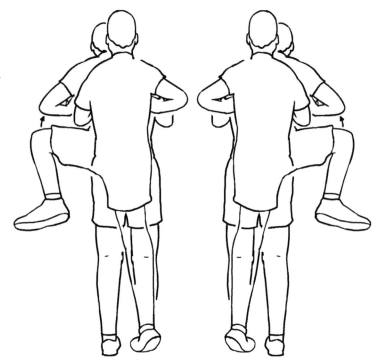

Begin with the basic push-up starting position. As you lower your body, lift your left foot off the ground and touch your left knee to your left elbow. Stop the movement once your chest is just above the ground and then push yourself back up returning your left foot to the starting position.

Repeat on the right side for the next rep and alternate left and right until you complete the set.

Useful tips for Spiderman push-ups:

It's best to do a few of the easier push-up variations as a warm-up before doing any of the superhero ones. These can also be done in a "decline" position by starting off with your feet on a chair. These are the toughest of the Spiderman variations and definitely only for the super-fit and strong.

1.5 Jump push-ups

Suitability: Super-fit.

Begin with the basic push-up starting position and lower your body until your chest is slightly off the ground. From this position, drive yourself up in an explosive movement so that your hands briefly lift off the ground as your elbows straighten. Catch yourself in a controlled manner as your hands again touch the floor, lowering yourself into the bottom position of the push-up. Repeat the movement to complete the next rep.

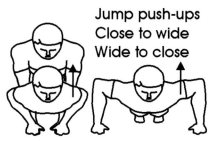

Jump push-ups
Close to wide
Wide to close

Useful tips for jump push-ups:

Jump push-ups are best done on a soft surface like a thick carpet. The velocity of the movement adds to the resistance on the push-up, intensifying the exercise significantly. You can also alternate the hand positions after each push-up, as illustrated in the diagram, so as to work each of the different muscles involved in the movement more intensely.

2. Squats

A squat is a phenomenal exercise. It strengthens the lower body and core providing a fantastic base of support for virtually all physical movements. It is also one of the best exercises for weight loss. Unfortunately, squats are generally believed to be a risky exercise, placing undue stress on the knees and back.

Now, there's no question that, when done incorrectly, squats can cause problems. But when the easier squat progressions are used and good form is maintained, these risks can be radically reduced. This means that you really don't need to be scared of this exercise. Do the movements the way they're supposed to be done and you can look forward to strengthening your body and enjoying the awesome benefits that this big exercise promises.

2.1 Full squats

Suitability: Intermediate, super-fit.
Stand with your feet hip-width apart and your arms by your sides. Lower your buttocks until you reach a spot where your thighs are parallel to the floor. As you bend down, extend your arms out in front of you to maintain good balance. With your weight on your heels, push yourself back into the starting position.

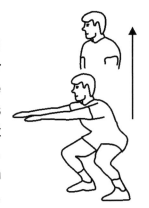

Useful tips for full squats:

One of the best ways to reduce the risk of injury is to squat with your body weight going backward rather than forward. This means that you should be able to "wiggle" your toes throughout the movement. If you feel any discomfort in your back or knees, don't squat as deep. Rather, begin with the super-shallow squat and progressively work your way toward doing the full ones.

As with all exercises, squats should be done with care and within the capability of the one doing them. If you cannot perform ten full squats in one go, then you must begin with the easier squat variations.

General variations for squats:

As with push-ups, there are two general variations to squats. These also involve different feet placements and timing. The variations can be applied to all the different squats and are suitable for all three fitness levels.

Feet placement for squat variation:

Similar to the hand placements for the push-ups, there are three different ways to position your feet doing squats:

- Hip-width apart
- Shoulder-width apart
- Wider than shoulder-width

Useful tips for feet placements:

It is best to have your toes pointing straight in front of you for the narrow stance, and for a wider stance to point them slightly outward to accommodate for hip rotation.

The closer your feet are together, the more the squat will work the front of your thighs (quads). As your feet get farther and farther apart, the more your inner thighs (adductors) are activated.

Timing for squat variation:

As I said with the push-ups, there are options for speed. Here are the two recommended for varying your squats:

- Regular: Two seconds down, one second up.
- Pause: Two seconds down with a two-second pause at the bottom.

Useful tips for timing:

Bending down slowly and rising more quickly is a great way to get more out of your squats. If you are strong enough, holding the position at the bottom for longer, say, five seconds, can add to the intensity of the movement.

Specific variations for squats:

There are four different squat progressions for you to choose from. The first three are suitable for all three fitness levels, but the forth one is only for the super-fit.

Easier squats:

- Super-shallow squats
- Wall squats
- Chair squats

More difficult squats:

- Jump squats

Let's take a closer look at each of them.

2.2 Super-shallow squats

Suitability: Beginner, intermediate.

The super-shallow squat is especially for beginners and those carrying excess weight. The idea is to use this minimal squat as a starting point for developing the strength necessary for doing the more difficult ones.

Begin as you would for a full squat with your back straight and feet hip-width apart. Contract your core muscles (abs) and lower your buttocks a little by bending your knees slightly. Return to an upright position keeping your weight on your heels, not your toes.

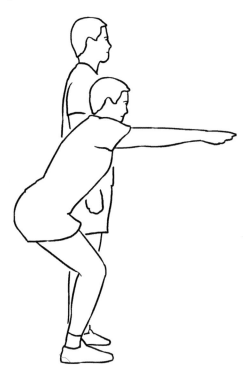

Useful tips for super-shallow squats:

Don't think for a moment that this squat is a waste of time; even the shallowest of dips can be useful. Simply dropping a little deeper each week will build strength safely. Remember, it's crucial that you're able to wiggle your toes throughout the movement. The "wiggle test" is your tool for making sure that you are squatting correctly.

2.3 Wall squats

Suitability: Beginner, intermediate.

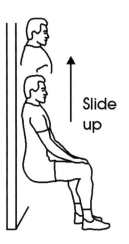

Slide up

With your feet hip-width apart and about a foot and a half away from the wall behind you, lean backward until your back is flat against the wall. From this position, slide your buttocks down the wall by bending your knees. Aim to lower yourself until your thighs are parallel with the floor. Hold for a count of two, and then press through your heels until your legs are again straight.

Useful tips for wall squats:

First things first, don't ever attempt this exercise on a rough wall; that's bound to turn out ugly. Having protected your clothes, let's turn our attention to doing the same for your body.

I prefer this exercise to be done with the upper body slightly away from the wall. That means only your buttocks rub on the wall through the movement. This keeps the weight in the heels and protects your back. If you're unable to pass the "wiggle test" throughout the movement, then you need to move your feet farther away from the wall to free up your toes and lessen any strain on your knees.

2.4 Chair squats

Suitability: Beginner, intermediate.

The chair squat naturally produces the backward movement that keeps the weight in the heels and protects the knees. That's why it's one of my favorites for beginners.

Start by standing the length of your foot in front of a stable chair, with your feet hip-width apart. Then sit back and as your buttocks touch the edge of the chair, stand up. It's that simple.

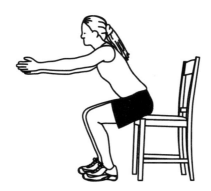

Useful tips for chair squats:

The height of the chair influences the degree of difficulty; the higher the chair, the less strenuous the exercise; the lower the chair, the harder it works you. If you can't find a chair that's high enough to suit you, a tall and stable table or a desktop will do. If you have particularly weak legs, then do the exercise as a "squat-sit." This means sitting back into the chair and standing up again with as little help from your arms as possible.

2.5 Jump squats

Suitability: Super-fit.

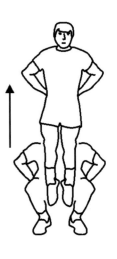

Begin as you would for a full squat with your feet hip-width apart and back straight. Lower your buttocks until you reach a spot where your thighs are parallel to the floor. With your weight on your heels and your arms out in front of you, jump up into the air pulling your hands back behind you. Make your landing as "soft" as possible by bending your knees as you land and pretending that you're coming down on a grape that you don't want to squash. Hold the low position of the squat for one second, and then repeat the jump and landing.

Useful tips for squat jumps:

Sean and I absolutely love jump squats. They produce great leg strength and can burn a whole load of calories. It's best, however, to save them for when you're on soft, carpeted floors or wearing supportive shoes to cushion your landing.

Jump squats are also useful for strengthening your calf muscles. A good way to get your calves working even harder is to do many shallow jump squats. This is a lot like skipping rope and can give you a super calf and cardio workout.

Moving to the core

There is no doubt in my mind that multiple short bouts of push-ups and squats done in a day are fabulous for your health and body shape. The versatility of these exercises makes them perfect for the warm-up, workout, and cool-down facets of your Spread-Workouts. By doing them regularly and progressing to the more challenging variations, you can look forward to developing your strength, coordination, and agility, which will make you look, feel, and function the way you want to.

In the next chapter, I'll discuss the three mid-section exercises we've chosen to build a solid bridge between your upper and lower body. But, before we get to those core exercises, I want to get you moving again.

Take a look back through this chapter and choose squat and push-up variations that you think are a safe fit for you right now. When you've done that, stand up and do ten reps of each if you are a beginner; twenty of each if you are an intermediate; and thirty of each if you are super-fit. When you are done with that, go grab a glass of water and move on to the next chapter.

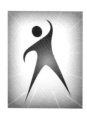

CHAPTER 4

The Core Triplet

Taking care of your stomach, back, buttocks, and sides

OVER THE PAST couple of years the core has become the center of attention amongst sportsmen, exercise professionals, and rehabilitation specialists. That's not because they are all interested in six-pack abs.

What has become abundantly clear is that a strong and stable mid-section is essential to higher performance, better balance, improved posture, and reduced risk of back injury. Without a solid bridge between the upper and lower body, physical function is impeded.

To help you develop the core muscles that make for good whole-body fitness, the 3-6-10 method uses a "core triplet" that includes:

1. Cross-leg crunches
2. Mantis extensions
3. Wall stick-ups

Together, these three exercises can work almost your entire mid-section. Your back, sides, buttocks, hip flexors, and "six-pack" all have to contract when you do the crunches, extensions, and stick-ups. The core triplet also does a great job of stretching tight muscles, which is good for maintaining flexibility.

As with the push-ups and squats, each individual core exercise has variations. One of the stand-out features of the variations is that they make it possible to do all three core exercises without having to lie down. This makes them ideal for use anywhere, anytime without having to concern yourself with a dirty floor.

There are obviously many other exercises like planks, bridges, hip lifts, and twists that can strengthen your core. Just because they are not included in the 3-6-10 plan doesn't mean you can't use them in your Spread-Workouts. In saying that, however, choosing to stick with the core triplet exercises will do more than enough to develop the kind of stomach, back, buttocks, and sides that look good and function well.

With that core thought, let's begin with cross-leg crunches.

1. Cross-leg crunches

Suitability: Beginner, intermediate, super-fit.

Something I love about this particular exercise is how well it *stretches* the glutes and *strengthens* the upper back and lower abs. This kind of stretch-strengthening effect is an essential component of developing optimal core stability and function.

This is how it's done: lie flat on your back with your knees bent. Hold your earlobes between your thumbs and forefingers, making sure that your elbows are pressed to the floor on either side of your head. Lift one leg and place the outer part of your ankle across the knee of your other leg. From this starting position, lift your shoulders and arms up off the floor, bringing your elbows together and your bent knee toward your elbows. Exhale forcefully through this part of the crunch movement. Return to the starting position by touching your elbows to the floor at the same time as the heel of your bent leg.

Remember to split the total number of reps you want to do equally between your left and right legs crossed.

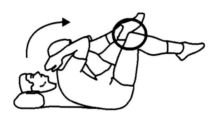

Useful tips for cross-leg crunches:

Putting your hands behind your head while doing this exercise will incline you to pull on your head, stressing your neck. This is why it's important to grab hold of your earlobes. If you feel like tugging on them, feel free.

To work the sides of your mid-section more specifically, try touching both elbows to the knee of your crossed leg. This will create a slight twisting movement and activate other important core muscles.

If lying on the floor isn't an option, you can use the standing variation called the "butterfly wing." This is how it's done: stand up straight, take hold of your earlobes, and press your elbows back. Lift your right knee and, at the same time, bring your elbows together to meet it. Exhale forcefully as you do this, and then return to the starting position. Repeat the movement by raising the left leg, then alternate left and right until you have completed your reps. The rhythmic movement of the elbows apart and then coming together should give the appearance of the opening and closing of a butterfly's wings.

This standing variation has a similar abdominal crunch effect to the one done lying down. It will also serve to strengthen your back and shoulders and stretch your chest. The downside is that the buttocks are not stretched as effectively as when the exercise is done lying on your back because there is no crossing of the legs. This is why a good mix of the lying down and standing versions is best.

2. Mantis extensions

Suitability: Beginner, intermediate, super-fit.
This fantastic exercise, otherwise known as the "bird dog," works the buttocks, back of the thighs, lower back, abs, and the front of the shoulders.

Begin on all fours supporting your weight on your hands and knees, keeping your back flat and your eyes facing the floor. Lift one arm straight out in front of you, and extend the leg of the opposite side straight behind you. Hold for a count of two, and then return to the all-fours position. Switch sides and repeat to complete your reps.

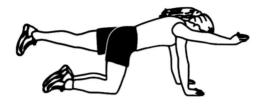

Useful tips for mantis extensions:

Working different parts of the shoulder and buttocks are possible by pointing your thumb and big toe in different directions through the movement. When you give a "thumbs up" with the raised hand, you work the front of your shoulder; giving a "thumbs down" works the back of it. Pointing the toes of your extended leg *inward* toward your other foot will work the middle part of your buttocks. Pointing your toes outward will work the outer part of it.

To do the standing version of this exercise, simply adopt the wall push-up starting position. Then take your right hand off the wall and point to the ceiling. At the same time, push your left heel backward, keeping your leg straight. It's imperative not to bend your knee. Hold the position for a count of two, and then return to the starting position. Repeat by alternating sides until you have completed your reps.

3. Wall stick-ups

Suitability: Beginner, intermediate, super-fit.

It's no secret that our "seated" lifestyles produce poor posture—chicken necks, hunched shoulders, hollow lower backs, and weak buttocks. Wall stick-ups are one of the best remedies, as they strengthen and stretch just about everything necessary to improve your overall posture.

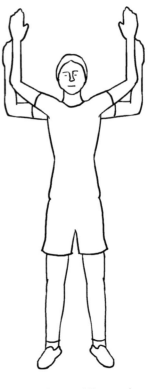

Start by leaning back against the wall with your hands in the air as if you were being held at gunpoint. Your elbows should be bent at 90° and your head, shoulders, elbows, hands, buttocks, and heels all touching the wall. From this starting position, forcefully breathe out while pulling in your belly button and trying to squeeze your lower back flat against the wall. At the same time, slide your hands up the wall as if you have been told to "stick 'em up higher." Be sure to keep your hands, elbows, shoulders, head, lower back, and buttocks as flat against the wall as possible throughout the movement. Hold the position for one to two seconds, and then relax back to the starting position as you breathe in.

Useful tips for wall stick-ups:

The most useful piece of advice I can give you about wall stick-ups is this: *do them every day*. You may find them difficult to do at first, because keeping everything against the wall is tough to do. If you do struggle, don't quit; keep working and they will get easier.

Rotating through the triplet

Now that each of the core-triplet exercises have been explained, the best way to use them is in *rotation*. If, for example, you have done cross-leg crunches as your first core exercise for the day, then do the mantis extensions and stick-ups for the second and third. If you do more core exercises in the day, then go back to the cross-leg crunches and repeat the cycle. Mixing things up like this hits the high notes of variety and produces balanced core strength.

To get a feel for how this works, I'd like you to think back to the push-up and squat variations that you chose to do at the end of the previous chapter. The plan is to do them again, but this time, with the core triplet in between. If you are a beginner, your short-bout rotation will look like this:

1. Ten push-ups
2. Six cross-leg crunches (three each side)
3. Ten squats
4. Six mantis extensions (three each side)
5. Ten push-ups
6. Five stick-ups
7. Ten squats

If you are intermediate or super-fit, do the same sequence but with the twenty reps of push-ups and squats and ten reps of each core exercise in between. These short bouts will probably take between two-and-a-half and three minutes. That's not a lot of time for something so good for you.

Breathing for better results

So, how did the set go?

Are the exercises you selected a good match for you? I hope so, but before you do any of them again, I want to draw your attention to another important aspect of your exercise—your *breathing*.

A proper breathing technique during each movement can make a big difference in your performance. The nice thing is that learning to breathe properly is straightforward. Simply get into the habit of following these three guidelines:

1. Breathe *in* through your nose and *out* through your mouth.
2. *Inhale* with the *relaxation* part of the movement.
3. *Exhale* with the *exertion* part of the movement.

For squats and push-ups, this means breathing *in* as you *lower* your body and breathing *out* as you rise *up* again. For the core triplet exercises, you breathe *out* when you bring your elbows to your knees in the crunch, lift your arm and leg in the mantis, and press everything against the wall in the stick-up. You then breathe *in* as you return to the starting position of each.

When you apply these principles you will quickly develop a good breathing rhythm for your exercises. Instead of hampering your performance by holding your breath, which is what most of us are inclined to do, you will deliver the necessary oxygen to your working muscles and clear the carbon dioxide from your bloodstream. This way you can enjoy even better results from your Spread-Workouts.

Summing up at the halfway mark

Before continuing with chapter 5, I think it's worth pausing for a quick review. What we know thus far is that exercise is really good for us. We also know that too many people are missing out on its benefits because they don't do enough of it. In the first chapter I suggested five reasons for the shortage. These I described as hurdles to exercise, and since that point have shown how four of these hurdles can be cleared by the 3-6-10 Spread-Workouts.

By re-packaging exercise into short bouts accumulated throughout the day, the *time* obstacle shrinks. The *difficulty* barrier is dismantled with super easy exercise progressions. Each exercise has been presented clearly, making the step over the *know-how* hurdle a small one. Because the 3-6-10 method uses only bodyweight exercises not requiring any specific place to perform, all your workouts are free and the *cost* encumbrance no longer exists.

The truth is that *your physical activity all adds up at the end of the day*, which leaves the all-or-nothing exercise mentality (and the handicaps that go with it) in the wake of more movement done more frequently and more conveniently than ever.

Now, feel free to move on.

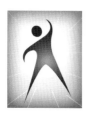

CHAPTER 5

Essential Exercise Principles

Everything you do either helps or hurts

HAVE YOU EVER thrown a ball into the air and expected it to remain there? I doubt it. Yet many people are inclined to think in zero-gravity ways when it comes to their health, fitness, and body shape. They start a new diet or gym program, do what's necessary for a short time, and then drift back to their old lifestyle, all the while assuming their results will stay.

But, as assuredly as what goes up must come down, your body responds to *all* that you do (and don't do). Sean and I like to say it like this: *Everything you do either helps or hurts in pursuit of your health and fitness goals*. It's what we call *The Law of Dynamic Impact* and it means that sustainable results only come from sustainable action.

The law also provides a great foundation for understanding two key exercise principles, namely, *reversibility* and *specificity*. A good grasp of these can make planning your workouts and interpreting your results much easier, so let's take a closer look at them.

Reversibility and continuity

The cruel reality is that muscles get smaller and fitness declines with inactivity. In as little as a week or two of no exercise, good conditioning can start coming undone. Possibly the worst thing about this *reversibility* is the disproportionate difficulty regaining the loss. Getting fit once you've lost it can be hard to do, which is why exercise *continuity* is crucial.

We already know from the first four exercise hurdles that exercising consistently is a challenge when single-session workouts are the only option. Even when you genuinely want to go to the gym, there are always reasons for not getting there. Leaving late from the office, an unexpected guest, or forgetting your workout clothes at home are only a few of the things that hurt. Regardless of the reasons, inconsistency is severely punished by reversibility.

Thankfully, with Spread-Workouts, it is entirely possible to maintain a high level of continuity even when these types of obstacles crop up. The worst-case scenario is that you might end up doing a little *less* than you had initially planned to do. But, remember, when every bit counts, less is infinitely better than *none* at all.

With each rep slowing down the rate of muscle and fitness loss, you can minimize the impact of reversibility. By enabling you to do reps so easily each day, week in and week out, Spread-Workouts lead to sustainable results. Their repetitive nature produces the all-important continuity that the sustainability we all want demands.

Specificity and cluster-sets

Tied in with the principle of reversibility is *specificity*. It's rather straightforward in that the particular muscles you exercise are the ones that get bigger and stronger. The muscles you fail to work are the ones that fail to develop.

In light of this, there is always the potential for training yourself into disproportion and dysfunction. Overtraining some parts and under-training others can make your body look funny and cause postural and functional imbalances. This is far from ideal, which is why it's vital that your Spread-Workouts engage your whole body by bundling the different 3-6-10 exercises together into *cluster sets*.

Getting a good mix of cluster sets, which include push-ups, squats, and one or more of the core exercises, is a great way to work the front, back, and sides of your upper body, as well as your lower body and buttocks. In the next chapter, I will tell you a whole lot more about how to do this. This way you can enjoy the benefits of a functionally well-balanced and proportional body.

A suitable warm-up

Sean and I both agree that a warm-up is important when working out. But with the typical 3-6-10 set lasting only a few seconds to a maximum of around five minutes, the traditional warm-up that increases heart rate, respiratory rate, and body temperature isn't necessary. What is needed is an approach that prepares and protects joints, ligaments, tendons, and muscles.

The great thing about each of the 3-6-10 exercises is that they are in and of themselves good warm-up movements. This means that there's no need for a separate warm-up routine. By simply beginning each new set *slowly* and by making good use of the easier exercise progressions, you can be suitably warmed up and reduce your risk of injury. What follows are two ways to do this.

Super-shallow starts

The first warm-up strategy is to begin each new set with super-shallow versions of each exercise. This means the first four, six, or even eight reps of each new exercise in your set should be only *halfway*. Take a push-up for example. You would lower your body only a portion of the way for the first few reps of a new set and then progress into the full movement as you feel comfortable to do so. The same "shallow" approach would apply to your squats and core exercises.

Exercise progressions

The second warm-up method is to work your way through various exercise progressions. Starting with a few wall push-ups or knee push-ups before doing regular push-ups would be a good example. Rotating through a few different progressions in your cluster sets builds up to the more adventurous and intense variations. These will ultimately have the greatest body-shaping effects.

When applied properly, the two warm-up methods I've

described are safe and effective. You will do well to get into the habit of using them in your Spread-Workouts.

Workout intensity

A crucial component of conditioning is getting the intensity right. While pushing yourself too hard can cause injury, not pushing yourself hard enough will fail to produce the results you want. In saying that, Sean and I always recommend a low intensity start to your Spread-Workouts. This means *limited reps* and *easy progressions* at first. Steadily upping the intensity as your body adapts is always better than doing too much too soon. All that usually means is injury and disruption to your workouts. That's why I will say it again: safety must come first.

Beyond the reduced injury risk of a low-intensity start, there are other advantages as well. Greater feelings of well-being and generally improved body function can occur within two to three weeks of doing small amounts of exercise. Better sleep, more energy, and sharper concentration are changes that people commonly describe. The body shaping gains are what take a little longer and demand the greatest intensity. In the long run, however, a slow and steady start wins both the health and shape races, so don't rush in.

Getting the intensity right is an individual thing. Choosing the total number of reps and exercise progressions that will be good for you when you start out will be easier with what comes next.

Number of reps per day

The best way to establish your starting number of reps is to use your current 3-6-10 fitness level. This is what you determined from your fitness estimation test in chapter 2. In the table below, find the recommendations for the total number of reps each fitness level should aim to do in a Spread-Workout day.

Beginner	100-200 reps
Intermediate	200-500 reps
Super-fit	>500 reps

I know Sean mentioned it in the introduction, but let me quickly clarify that when I talk about a "rep" I am referring to a single complete movement of an exercise. The "total" number, therefore, is the sum of *every* rep of *all* the exercises done in a day.

In Sean's and my experience, these "total rep" starting points are good ones. However, after a few days of doing your own Spread-Workouts, you will be in a position to make adjustments. Whether it be up or down, do whatever you feel will fit best.

Personal goals

Your personal goals are the next thing to consider in your decision. Not everybody is after the same thing, so if your goal is to get fitter and lose weight, then you will need to focus on doing *as many reps* as you can each day. If your goal is to be well toned and build muscle, then focus on doing the *more difficult exercise* progressions. You will probably need to experiment a bit and fine-tune things every two weeks or so based on how your body is responding. This means that you need to stay in touch by gathering feedback.

Keeping score, as it were, is quite easy to do. You don't need much more than a tape measure to record changes in your waist, hips, arms, and thighs. This can be done every week or two. In addition to your measurements, I recommend taking pictures of yourself every two to four weeks. This should be long enough between shots for you to see the comparative differences and be motivated by the change.

Please don't stop short at measuring only appearance, though. How you are feeling in response to the Spread-Workouts is also important to consider. Recognizing that you have more energy, for example, can be a great catalyst for maintaining continuity and even upping your intensity.

Putting reps and progressions together

Now, let's get practical and, in two steps, translate all of what's gone before into a number and an exercise list for you to begin with.

1. Take a moment to look at the reps table again. When you're done, write down how many reps you are going to start with.

   Reps per day: _____

2. Take a few minutes to go back to chapters 3 and 4 and review the different exercises. Compile a list of the push-ups, squats, and core exercises that you want to use.

Push-ups: _____

_____

Squats: _____

_____

Core triplet: _____

_____

Great, now, let's slow down and touch on one more important exercise principle...

Rest and recovery

So far I have highlighted the need for exercise continuity and balanced workouts, as well as addressed the value of a warm-up and the right Spread-Workout intensity. What's just as important for me to do is underline the key role of rest.

Proper rest is essential for recovery and improving health, fitness, and strength. Suitable breaks between sets and between days give the body the time it needs to replenish its energy, and to repair muscles, ligaments, and tendons. The time out also makes room for adaptation of the nervous and circulatory systems.

The nice thing with Spread-Workouts is that the rest between sets is automatically taken care of. With anything from a few minutes to two hours between each set, your body has more than enough time to recover. The only other thing you need to do to rest properly is take a day off once a week. What I suggest is that you make it the last day of your week. This will give you the time you need to recover well and will also contribute to developing a good rhythm and routine, something we'll consider more closely in the next chapter.

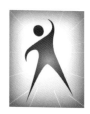

CHAPTER 6

Setting the Tone

Linked sets, a flying start,
and a dash of improvisation

FORMULATING A GOOD routine for your Spread-Workouts is a good idea; it enables you to keep your exercise flowing through the day. To help you structure your workouts, it's useful to consider *how many* short-bout sets you will aim for a day, *when* you will do them, and *what* those sets might include.

Sets per day

The number of sets you use to accumulate your reps in a day is ultimately up to you. When making your decision, though, it's helpful to factor in the *total number of reps* you've chosen to do along with your *personal schedule*.

I suggest that, to begin with, your Spread-Workouts are made up of a *minimum* number of sets based on your fitness level and the guidelines for the reps from the previous chapter:

- Beginner: 100-200 reps in 3-4 sets
- Intermediate: 200-500 reps in 3-6 sets
- Super-fit: 500 or more reps in 4-6 sets

As I said, these are the minimum number of sets you should aim to do a day. Having *more* short bouts of exercise rather than less is better. Remember, long periods of sedentary behavior are dangerous, so breaking them up with frequent movement start-ups offers additional benefit.

In terms of your personal schedule, if you are busy and only have a few seconds or a minute for each set, then you will naturally need to split your total reps into more sets. As I've already indicated, that's actually a good thing.

Make your choice

Okay, with reps and schedule in mind, how many sets are you going to start out with? When you have an idea, write it down.

I'm going to begin my Spread-Workouts with _____sets per day.

Great, now let's consider the *timing* of those sets.

When is it best to do your sets?

One of the best things about Spread-Workouts is there's never a "wrong" time to exercise. Any gap you have in your day, planned or otherwise, is an opportunity to get moving. In saying that, however, I do think that having a mix of *planned (linked)* and *opportunist (in-betweener)* sets is wise. Let me explain.

Linked sets

No matter how variable somebody's schedule, there are always things that are the same, such as waking up, brushing teeth, going to work, arriving home, and going to bed. These relatively fixed things are useful for creating *exercise links*. By piggybacking sets on habits you already have, you can create an *immediate exercise habit* and add *structure* to your Spread-Workouts. When your existing habits become the triggers for your new exercise plan (which you have no excuse not to do) you automatically start moving.

Think about it. If brushing your teeth and going to bed prompted you to do ten push-ups, ten squats, and ten of one of the core exercises, assuming you brush twice, that's ninety reps routinely accounted for each day. Add another ten of each to arriving at work and arriving home from work and the rep count jumps to 150. Done in five sets, the frequency of movement is also heading in the right direction. Not bad and not difficult, don't you think?

Linked sets don't need to be long, although I do think it's a good idea to fill them up. Doing twenty of each as an intermediate, in the same pattern I just described, will mean three hundred reps a day. Make that thirty of each if you are super-fit, then 450 reps are accounted for. By making these habit-attached sets the fullest ones, it's possible to *consistently* get through the bulk of your reps every day. That's why linked sets are a vital component of successful Spread-Workouts.

In-betweeners

As you get into the swing of accumulating your exercise, you will no doubt find more gaps in your day. Some of those gaps will be too short to do full cluster sets. But, that's no problem at all. Due to the fact that every bit counts you can take advantage of any gap that presents itself. Doing only a few reps of even a single exercise in-between your other things is absolutely fine and something we encourage you to do often.

Be sure to mix things up well, though. If your first in-betweener set was mostly an upper body one, then try to make your next set a lower body or a core one. This helps to maintain good balance.

Collectively, the in-betweeners and linked sets establish the *timing* of your daily short bouts. Together they will, most likely, fit something like this:

- A set linked to waking up
- In-betweeners (1-2)
- A set linked to lunch (before)
- In-betweeners (1-2)
- A set linked to bedtime

This is an ideal Spread-Workout.

A flying start

Before moving on to the third aspect of the 3-6-10 sets, I want to take a moment to point out the value of a good start to the day. There's no question that getting off to a *flying* start promotes more successful Spread-Workouts. That's because the morning usually establishes the tone for the rest of the day.

It's really a mind thing. You see, when you get going well, the inclination is to avoid undoing the good work with a poor follow-through. So, you keep pushing. It's as if the motivation to build on the foundation improves and awareness of opportunities to add sets throughout the day is heightened.

With a flying start being such a good thing, here are three suggestions for how many reps to include in a strong starting set:

- Beginners: Thirty to sixty reps.
- Intermediates: Sixty to ninety reps.
- Super-fit: One hundred to one hundred and fifty reps.

A flying start to the day usually means a flying finish. You will not go wrong by committing to making this the most important set of your day.

Formatting your sets

Okay, let's get back to discussing the 3-6-10 sets in terms of what they might look like. In other words, let's talk about the *format*.

Not all of your sets will be the same. That's a given. Depending on where you are, how much time you have, and what you are wearing, you might use different exercises in different orders and do a different number of reps. To help you think through the variables, I think it's useful to give you three basic formats to consider. When you have a feel for what your options are you can then make your decisions as you see fit.

I'll begin with the all-inclusive one, the *RPC format*.

1. RPC format

RPC stands for *Rotation Progression Cluster*. It's the big daddy of the cluster set. It may sound complicated, but the name actually reveals the intention and structure, which is to *rotate* through *various progressions* of *all three basic exercises*. Here's an example that I'd like you to try. It's actually for the intermediates and super-fit, so, if you are a beginner, I suggest you half the reps and stick with the easier progressions through each rotation.

1st Rotation:

- Ten super-shallow squats
- Ten super-shallow push-ups
- Ten stick-ups

2nd Rotation:

- Twenty full squats
- Twenty regular push-ups
- Twenty mantis extensions

3rd Rotation:

- Ten squat jumps
- Ten Spiderman push-ups
- Ten cross-legged crunches

The advantage of these RPC sets is that they work the whole body and include a warm-up for the more demanding progressions at the end. This makes them perfect for your longer sets, preferably the ones linked to your daily habits.

2. Target format

Sets based on the target format are ones that work the smaller, weaker parts of the body more specifically. These sets are especially useful for correcting imbalances in shape, strength, and function. If, for example, you feel that your legs are underdeveloped from all the sitting that you do at the office, then including sets that concentrate on exercising your lower body is a good idea.

As with most things in the 3-6-10, the target sets can be done in more ways than one. You can target specific parts by doing more reps, using more intense exercise progressions, or a combination of the two. This last option is most effective.

Just remember, it is best to do the progressions that are appropriate to your fitness level to begin with. As you get stronger and fitter, you can progress to the more advanced variations. I will say it again, safety is the first priority.

Another thing to consider is combining the target and RPC formats. These *target rotation progression cluster sets* (a mouthful, I know) look something like this:

1st Rotation:

- Ten super-shallow squats
- Twenty super-shallow push-ups
- Ten stick-ups

2nd Rotation:

- Ten full squats
- Twenty regular push-ups
- Ten mantis extensions

3rd Rotation:

- Five squat jumps

- Ten Spiderman push-ups
- Five cross-legged crunches

These hybrid sets can also be done *without* the rotation. Here's an example of one, again, for the super-fit category:

- Twenty super-shallow squats
- Ten super-shallow push-ups
- Twenty regular push-ups
- Ten jump push-ups
- Twenty stick-ups

Depending on how much you want to strengthen and shape a particular part of your body, you can vary the number of target cluster sets you include in a workout day. You can do a few or a lot, or even do all of your sets this way until you have achieved your goal. Again, it's totally up to you.

By using the various principles from the previous chapter and the different set options from this one, you should be able to create a great Spread-Workout program; one that puts your health, shape, and fitness goals well within your reach.

3. Improvisation format

Okay, I'll admit that calling this third format a format is a contradiction. It's a bit like saying the only consistent thing about someone is their inconsistency. You see, in the improvisation format, *anything goes.* So, the format is that *there is no format,* which makes room for complete Spread-Workout flexibility.

License to improvise allows you to overcome most restrictions in ways that the other formats don't. When time permits only a few reps, or things like clothing or the immediate environment get in the way of doing particular exercises, knowing that you can do *anything in any quantity* enables you to fill the gaps for maximum results.

A tight uniform, for example, might make doing regular squats nearly impossible, but the same uniform could still make way for wall push-ups and stick-ups. A dirty floor is a legitimate reason not to do regular push-ups, but it doesn't get in the way of squats. Similarly, you might really be pushed for time, but how long does it take to do ten quick push-ups? Not long, I assure you.

Here are four examples of improvisation sets and how long they took me to do in between writing this:

1. Five stick-ups: eight seconds (no pause at the top)
2. Ten regular squats: twelve seconds
3. Five super-shallow push-ups, ten regular push-ups, five jump push-ups: twenty-five seconds
4. Thirty push-ups and thirty cross-leg crunches: seventy seconds

Let's be serious, I doubt there's anybody who cannot find gaps of ten, twenty, thirty, or even seventy seconds in their day. In fact, I am convinced that when you start looking, you are going to find periods of one, two, and even three minutes in which you can do a whole lot more than you currently do. But whether you have the time to do longer sets or the location to do all three exercises or not, improvisation sets make Spread-Workouts possible for everybody. All you need to be is awake.

Now, there is one more thing about the improvisation format (non-format), that I want to tell you about. It has to do with that all-or-nothing mentality that notoriously gets in the way of conventional, single-session workouts. I know from personal experience that the thought of having to do progression-rotation cluster sets can be a hindrance. These sets require a bit more time and an environment that's friendly to all the exercises, so it's easy for them to seem too big, inconvenient, or even impossible. All-or-nothing can easily put a stop to your Spread-Workouts when the thinking is if the "whole thing" can't be done there's no point doing any of it. This is where the freedom to improvise can keep your Spread-Workouts on track. Just because a given number of reps can't be done in the time available, or a particular exercise is obstructed by circumstances, there's no reason to miss out on adding something. Never forget that the heartbeat of the Spread-Workout is *every movement counts*. If you keep this in mind, you will keep the path clear of the all-or-nothing exercise killer.

"Nobody made a greater mistake than he who did nothing because he could only do a little." –Edmund Burke

So much from so little

This novel approach to exercise offers so much and demands so little. Despite having only five basic exercises, the 3-6-10 Health and Body Shaper's variations and progressions along with the different set formats provide plenty of options for you to personalize your Spread-Workouts.

Just remember, start slowly. Take your first week to get into the swing of things using the time to get comfortable with the exercises and to sharpen your awareness of opportunities throughout your day. Look carefully and you will spot one right now.

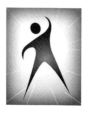

CHAPTER 7

Maximizing Your Results

The number ten, a professional secret, and a neat idea

MAXIMIZATION IS A CONCEPT that we are all familiar with. It's the idea of getting the most out of something, preferably as economically as possible. It's how our minds are wired to work. To help you get the most out of your Spread-Workouts, which is something Sean and I want for you, I have included three things that we think will help:

1. The ten-target
2. Periodization
3. Non-Exercise Activity Thermogenesis (NEAT)

Each is quite different from the other, but together they will go a long way in giving you the biggest return on your movement investment.

The ten-target

A great way to get great results is with an extra push. Safely doing that little bit more can make the difference between good health and better health, good shape and great shape. One way of doing this is *aiming for ten.* Ten is such a complete number and therefore a logical target to want to reach. Arriving at ten gives the feeling of completion, which is naturally motivating. The idea is to aim to finish your reps in batches of ten. If, for example, you've done one, then try to do ten. If you have done eleven, then go for twenty. Doing this can take you further in your Spread-Workouts than you otherwise might have gone.

To ensure that you always reach your ten-target, you must learn to *change gears.* By this I mean using your easier exercise progressions to get through. If, for example, you have reached seventeen push-ups and feel you just can't do anymore, you can gear down by dropping to your knees to finish the last three with knee push-ups. The same applies for the squats and core exercises. By using this nifty trick, you will find yourself doing more and enjoying greater success.

On top of the health and body-shaping benefits of aiming for ten, an added bonus is gaining mastery over yourself. Learning not to stop short of your goal, but to push through until you reach it will develop your self-control. This is, without a doubt, the most important character quality for any successful change.

In short, the ten-target gives you something higher to aim for, and when you shoot higher, you're bound to hit higher. I'd say that's ten out of ten, wouldn't you?

Periodization

Well-timed pushes and breaks produce special results. Ask any serious athlete and he will tell you that a progressive increase in exercise load mixed with proper rest periods is highly effective for improving conditioning. He'll say that in order to reach the highest highs in performance, he has to *periodize* his training.

Any athlete who attempts to go flat-out full time will find himself flat on his back in no time. That's why getting the balance between exercise and rest right, which is what periodization basically is, is vital for peak performance and longevity in sport. It's something the elite sportsmen all know about, yet it's foreign to most people wanting to improve their health, lose weight, and get into better shape. You might not be familiar with it either. The problem is that not periodizing your training properly is likely to see you hurt yourself or land you up on the quitters' heap. Neither is ideal.

Most fitness professionals don't bother telling their clients about periodization. They either work it into their clients' programs without their knowledge, which is fine, or, more commonly, they don't say anything about it because they're not expecting those clients to get much beyond a few weeks on the program. Sean and I think you will go a lot longer with this one. I already mentioned that continuity is easier to achieve with Spread-Workouts. That's why we anticipate your new exercise plan being one you keep doing and why we want you to factor in this professional secret.

The way to go about periodizing is easy. All you need to do is arrange your Spread-Workouts into a ten-week program as follows:

- Weeks 1-2: Low intensity
- Weeks 3-4: Moderate intensity
- Weeks 5-6: High intensity
- Weeks 7-8: Moderate intensity
- Week 9: Highest intensity
- Week 10: Rest week

The varying intensities relate mainly to the reps. The idea is to start off low for the first two weeks, and then increase them over weeks three and four, and then increase again in weeks five and six. In weeks seven and eight there is an easing off to the same level as in weeks four and five. Then there is a sharp increase for week nine, which is followed by a rest week.

The number of reps you adjust by each time is variable. It might be as few as ten or twenty per day, or as many as a hundred. Again, this is totally up to you. Simply let your current fitness level and goals help you decide. From there, if you follow the ups and downs in the weeks as I have described them, you will do enough to mix things up in a way that is good for you.

You can also periodize your workouts by using the different exercise progressions. If you choose to do this, you can still use the same pattern as for the reps. For instance, in weeks one and two, you might do wall push-ups, while in weeks three and four you do knee push-ups. In weeks five and six, you do regular push-ups. In weeks seven and eight, you go back to knee push-ups, and in week nine, you do the more intense, Spiderman push-ups. It's rather straightforward.

Please note that all intensity increases, whether they are in reps, progressions, or a combination of the two, should be kept small and based on your improving strength and fitness. This is essential to doing things safely.

Getting personal

Something Sean and I have always agreed upon is to only ever advise others to do things that we would be willing to do if we were in their same situation. Whether it's a test, a medication, a supplement, or a lifestyle change, we make a point of doing as we say. As you know, Spread-Workouts are no exception.

Depending on where we are, though, we don't always stick to equipment-free training. We often use different things like physio balls, medicine balls, dumbbells, bands, TRXs, pull-up bars, and Bosus as we accumulate our exercise through the day. These various tools provide great variety and keep things fresh. In saying that, there are still days when we stick purely to the 3-6-10 approach. When we do, this is what they look like:

Ryan's day: 610 reps

Time	Squats	Push-ups	Core	Minutes
7:10 a.m.	10	10	10	0:40
7:25 a.m.	50	50	50	4:55
11:40 a.m.	50	50	50	4:49
1:50 p.m.	30	---	10	1:15
4:58 p.m.	50	50	50	4:29
8:50 p.m.	30	50	10	2:25
TOTALS	220	210	180	18:33

Sean's day: 612 reps

Time	Squats	Push-ups	Core	Minutes
9:00 a.m.	20	20	12	2:15
9:20 a.m.	30	30	30	2:13
10:28 a.m.	15	15	15	1:29
12:00 p.m.	30	30	15	2:45
1:12 p.m.	20	20	10	2:13
2:38 p.m.	50	20	20	2:59
5:23 p.m.	50	50	20	3:27
10:47 p.m.	30	30	30	2:19
TOTALS	245	215	152	19:40

On average, whether we use equipment or not, we get through between four hundred and seven hundred reps in a Spread-Workout. This means that we spend a minimum of between twelve and twenty-two minutes exercising a day.

I need to add that Spread-Workouts aren't the only thing we do. But we certainly get to do a whole lot more than we otherwise would if we relied only on our longer, single-session workouts. Like everyone else, we can find it difficult to fit a thirty- to sixty-minute workout into the day. Admittedly, there are also other times when we just don't feel like it.

When those low states of no get-up-and-go press down on us, the shear convenience of our Spread-Workouts comes to the rescue. A cluster set of fifty squats, fifty push-ups, and fifty core exercises is something that, no matter how flat we feel, we just cannot justify putting off. The result is that we end up accumulating exercise and enjoying the benefits of it even in our worst times.

At the end of the day, this exercise accumulation strategy is one that works wonders for us and we are super confident that it can do the same for you. That's why we gladly recommend it.

A NEAT idea and a hot combination

Seeing as this book is not merely aimed at using movement to produce fitter and stronger bodies, but also to help with weight loss, I must point out the benefits of *non-exercise activity thermogenesis* (NEAT).

What's become abundantly clear through the research of Dr. James Levine of the Mayo Clinic is that everyday things like standing, dancing, running around in the garden with kids, taking out the garbage, and carrying the groceries to and from the car are significant contributors to energy expenditure. In other words, you can burn a lot more calories each day by spending more time on your feet.

In their book *Move a Little, Lose a Lot,* Dr. James Levine and Selene Yeager suggest that, "Our current obesity and related health woes stem from the fact that modern life in the Internet-driven electronic age has increasingly leeched NEAT from our existence to the tune of up to 1,500 to 2,000 calories a day."[5]

When you look at those figures, you don't need to be a genius to see the implications for weight loss. In fact, in *Move a Little, Lose a Lot*, there are examples of people losing forty, fifty, and even sixty-plus pounds after adopting a NEAT-activated lifestyle. Simple things like parking farther from your office building or walking to work, taking the stairs instead of the elevator, and having your meetings walk-and-talk style can make a big difference. The fat bottom line is that becoming a "high-NEAT-worth" individual is a practical way to support the weight loss benefits of your exercise.

A great way to ensure you do more non-exercise activity is to use what we call the "NEAT-Q." The NEAT-Q is a question to ask yourself whenever you're about to sit down. "Do I really need to sit in order to perform this task?" If the answer is yes, and I mean a legitimate yes, then feel free to sit. But if the answer is no, then make a point of standing; better yet, walk around.

Just think about it. If you go through your day asking this question every time you're on the phone, how much time will you spend either standing or pacing around? Probably a lot more than you currently do, right? I suspect so. Now, say you made the NEAT-Q a habit with other things like reading the paper, watching the news, drinking your tea or coffee, and taking the bus (metro), wouldn't it help you increase the amount of energy you burn in a day? I'm sure it would, which is why if you want to lose weight, the NEAT-Q must become something you ask yourself regularly.

By combining the NEAT-Q with your 3-6-10 Spread-Workouts, you end up with a hot combination. It's an *equipment-free system* that's convenient, flexible, and inexpensive. It can work your upper body, lower body, and core and contribute to a significant increase in calorie burn. All together this leads to a well-balanced body that looks, feels, and functions better.

Neat, don't you think?

More opportunities for us to stand and move

In light of what you've read, my suggestion is that, from this point until the end of the book, you read standing. Whether you have it in print or a digital version, I am convinced that's doable.

Also, before we get to the end of this chapter, let's both take a break and do a quick set. I'll make it a short one and, this time, add a few variations:

- Wall push-ups with hands placed close together. This targets the back of the arm (triceps) more specifically.
- Shallow squats done with a two-second pause at the bottom.
- Regular push-ups with hands placed far apart (wide hand push-up).
- Regular squats to be done with feet placed farther apart in order to target the inner thighs (adductors), and a two-second pause at the bottom to add to the intensity.

If you don't like the variations I've suggested, feel free to try any others that you might prefer.

Beginner:
- Ten wall push-ups
- Ten shallow squats
- Five stick-ups

Intermediate and super-fit:
- Twenty regular push-ups
- Twenty regular squats
- Ten stick-ups

Okay, let's get going and then come back to finish up with the final chapter where Sean will take over and get practical.

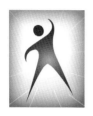

CHAPTER 8

Everything You Need

*Confirmations, opportunities,
and the final hurdle*

BY THIS STAGE, Ryan has given you almost everything you need to get moving. To ensure that you get off to the best possible start, I want to guide you through four final preparation steps:

1. Confirmation of your fitness level and exercise choices.
2. Confirmation of your starting number of reps and sets.
3. Becoming an exercise opportunist.
4. Reminders and tips to round things off.

By the time I'm done, you will have the complete picture and everything you need for the best possible Spread-Workout results.

1. Confirm your fitness level and exercise choices

Can you confirm your current 3-6-10 fitness level, and have you decided on which of the exercise progressions and variations are the best fits for you? If your answer is yes, then you can move on. If you aren't yet sure about either your fitness level or the exercises to begin with, then go back to page 16 and do the fitness estimation test. Then review chapters 3 and 4 and decide on your exercises. When you know where you fit into the 3-6-10 approach, then you are ready to move on.

2. Confirm your number of starting reps and sets

In chapter 5 you had the opportunity to decide on the number of reps you'd like to start off with. Confirm that you are happy with this number. If you aren't, then adjust it until you are. Once you've done that, also confirm the basic number of sets that you are aiming for each day. This need not be fixed, but it's good to have a number in mind to keep you moving steadily through the day.

3. Become an exercise opportunist

When starting out with the 3-6-10 plan it is important to train yourself to spot exercise opportunities. In conjunction with the sets that you have linked to your daily habits, it's the opportunist ones that add spice to your Spread-Workouts.

To get your thoughts going, here are twenty different opportunities that I can think of. The list is far from exhaustive, but it's a good place to start as you think about ones you might have in your own day.

The first

First thing after getting out of bed in the morning is the ideal time for a short cluster of the easier progressions. This set is the one that stretches you and gets you moving.

The loosener

Before a morning shower is a great time to drop in a set of the lighter exercises. This set can take the stretch to the next level of "looseness."

The starter

Directly after a refreshing morning shower is the ideal time for the *flying start*. Two to four minutes is long enough to move you through a good number of reps, and short enough not to get you all sweaty. Whether the flying start is linked to getting out of the shower or not, I think this set is an absolute must for every Spread-Workout day.

The breakfast-breezer

The thirty or more seconds spent waiting for things like the toaster to pop or the blender to mix your morning smoothie provide an ideal time for a three-by-ten or three-by-twenty cluster set.

The first good-bye

As you're about to leave for work you have the opportunity to throw in a "good-bye" set. Even if it is just a few stick-ups, this is a good one to get into the habit of doing.

The work hello

One of the best things to do on arriving at work is to run through a medium intensity set of ten to thirty reps of each exercise. This two-minute session is perfect to do while waiting for your computer to start up and your e-mails to come through.

The T-easer

If you are in the habit of drinking tea or coffee through the day, then a quick three-by-ten set to ease you into each cup is perfect.

The meeting mover

When you have a meeting scheduled it's good to do ten of each exercise before it begins. If you are inclined to be anxious speaking in meetings or doing presentations, then you can look forward to the added benefit of the calming effect that this set can offer.

The lucky lunchtime

If you are fortunate enough to have a lunch break, then this is an opportunity to add a linked set into the middle of your day. Give this one an extra push, and then sit down and enjoy your meal.

The phone shaper

Doing a short set, like ten squats, after each phone call is a helpful way to shape your thoughts and body at the same time. It also adds to the NEAT benefits of having stood or walked around while on the phone.

The second good-bye

Leaving work for the day provides a wonderful opportunity to do an intense set. With no worries about how you look, this is a time to let your hair down and do twenty or more of each exercise as a farewell to the office.

The second hello

One of the best ways to get rid of tension that built up at the office is to do another two- to four-minute cluster set on arriving home. Make this a well balanced one and rotate through three or more sets of ten of each exercise. Build up the intensity by doing more challenging progressions as you get through each cycle of ten.

The ad ace

If you are someone who watches TV, the commercial breaks provide a super opportunity to exercise. Simply cycle through sets of ten to twenty of each exercise until your show starts again. Do this one consistently and you will soon be converting ads to abs!

The score

If you are a sports fan then it's time to get off the sideline and into the game. Commit to doing the exercises that target areas you want to shape most each time your team scores or something exciting happens. These can often turn into serious workouts and add to your Spread-Workout score.

Child's play

If you have children, then be sure to include them in your Spread-Workouts. In our experience, by the time we hit the floor for the push-ups, Ryan's daughters, Donna (6) and Hannah (3), are either on our backs or lying on the floor next to us and ready to go themselves. Even Kelsey, who is now only seven months, is included at times. These "family" sets are often the most fun, and the benefits extend to everyone involved. For obvious reasons we recommend that any "child's play" set be done as an improvisation set so that you can go with the flow and the mood of the moment.

The social set

There is often an opportunity to exercise in casual social gatherings. The next time you are sitting around chatting with your friends, ask them how fit they think they are. Tell them that you have a five-minute fitness estimation test that they can use to find out. Then take the opportunity to demonstrate it. If they decide not to do the test, that's okay—you at least got to do the set that you wanted to.

Partner up

If you are with someone who is also keen on doing more exercise, then get them to do sets with you whenever you are together. Partnering up can provide that extra motivation and is something I strongly recommend.

Swimmer's set

The next time you go for a swim do ten or more squat jumps in the pool. This is an ideal place to do them, especially if you are just starting out with this intense progression of the exercise.

Ex-smoker's break

If you are a smoker, then this is my chance to encourage you to quit the filthy habit and replace your smoke breaks with good, clean exercise.

The last

The best way to finish your day is to finish strong. Doing a set of the more challenging exercises before bed is bound to add shape to both your body and your day. Going to bed is another one of those daily habits that lends itself to a linked set. If, however, you struggle to fall asleep afterward, then don't do this one. A good night's rest is the better option.

After reading through my top twenty, I'm sure you can picture yourself doing some, if not all, of them. If you can think of any other opportunities to build exercise sets into your day, then be sure to use them too. Remember, working exercise into and around your schedule is about *taking* opportunities as well as *making* them. As Orison Swett Marden said, "Don't wait for extraordinary opportunities. Seize common occasions and make them great. Weak men wait for opportunities. Strong men make them."

I'm challenging you to be strong.

4. Reminders and tips for the best results

To round things off, I want to give you ten tips that will help you get the most out of your 3-6-10 Spread-Workouts. These are mostly reminders of things already covered in the book or are otherwise common sense. By implementing these you can look forward to the best possible results.

1. Drink a full glass of water after each exercise set. This exercise-water link will ensure good hydration and better health.

2. Include two to three fixed times for cluster sets each day. A good spread across morning, afternoon, and evening would be ideal.

3. Create reminders for yourself to do your sets throughout the day. Forgetfulness is a real threat to the successful application of Spread-Workouts.

4. Keep note of your sets. By writing down what you have done, you can remind yourself of what still needs to be done and even motivate yourself to do more.

5. Spread-Workouts needn't be your only form of exercise. Neither should you feel restricted to doing only the exercises in this book. If you want to improve your endurance, then it's a good idea to do two or more longer, single-session workouts a week. Also, if you want to develop a specific part of your body that you feel the 3-6-10 exercises aren't targeting sufficiently, then include other resistance exercises that will. I recommend upper body "pulling" exercises such as chin-ups, pull-downs, and rows as examples of what you can include.

6. A good exercise breathing technique is an easy way to improve your results. You can go back to the end of chapter 4 if you need a reminder of what to do.

7. Sore muscles deserve rest. This doesn't mean no exercise, but rather resting those muscles that are particularly tender by doing exercises that engage them less.

8. Use the 3-6-10 warm-up methods when starting any new set that includes the difficult progressions. The same

applies if you begin a set after sitting for longer than two hours.

9. Do as many RPC sets as you can. By working through the exercises in reps of ten with each new cycle being a more difficult progression, you can increase the intensity of your workouts for the best body-shaping results.

10. If weight loss is your goal, then you must increase your non-exercise activity (NEAT) and follow an appropriate eating plan. I like to summarize eating for weight loss like this:

- Eat less
- Eat more home-prepared meals
- Eat mostly simple, whole foods like fruit and vegetables (raw whenever possible)
- Eat slowly
- Go organic if you have the choice

If you follow these basic guidelines, you will succeed at achieving your goal.

The fifth hurdle

In chapter 1, Ryan identified five hurdles to exercise. In chapter 4, he explained how four of those can be cleared with Spread-Workouts. By this stage you are sufficiently equipped to use the 3-6-10 approach to overcome those four. All that remains to address is the final hurdle: "I don't like to exercise."

If this is what stands in your way, then think about this: Not everything we like is good for us, and not everything that's good for us is what we like. That's life. Not everyone loves doing their job, but they do it anyway; they know what's best for them. No work means no roof over their heads, clothes on their backs, or food in their mouths. In other words, they act in line with their better judgement rather than their impulsive desires.

When it comes to health, the same self-control should apply. That's because few things compare with how exercise protects and enhances well-being. I urge you to exercise more of it. At least be willing to try out the 3-6-10 Spread-Workout approach. It doesn't get more convenient than this. If you do, I am sure that you will actually learn to enjoy the rewards of looking, feeling, and functioning better. Like it or not, a dislike for exercise should never be a big enough obstacle to keep you from its many benefits.

With that in mind, I encourage you to *get over it* and join us on the path to anytime, anywhere, equipment-free exercise for better health and greater shape. It really is doable and it really is worth it.

Let's move!

*"A decision today changes tomorrow forever." –**John Di Lemme***

ПО SШEAT

No Obstacles Spread-Workout Exercise Accumulation Training

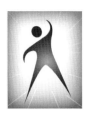

APPENDIX A

Shirts, Skirts, and Ties

A POTENTIAL OBSTACLE to applying the 3-6-10 Health and Body Shaper is restrictive clothing. Shirts, skirts, ties, suits, high heels, and pointy shoes can make things more difficult. If this is something that you have to contend with, then here are three suggestions that might help.

1. Test all the exercise variations and progressions to see which ones are still possible when you are in uniform. Wall push-ups, super-shallow squats, and stick-ups are usually doable in even the most limiting clothing. If these are the only exercises you can do that's fine; at least do them.

2. Do the bulk of your Spread-Workouts when you are not in "uniform." This would include doing as many reps as you can before and after you suit up.

3. Switch your rest day. Unless you work seven days a week, this would mean choosing to have your rest day when you are most restricted by your clothes. Then, on

the full day without any clothing restrictions, work extra hard and accumulate reps for the week.

The reality is that restrictive clothing is a challenge, but it's not one that makes exercise impossible. At least do what you can when you're "tied up," and make up for lost reps when you're "free." This way you can even look better in uniform.

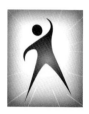

APPENDIX B

Look Out

THERE COMES A POINT where any task can seem too big. When this happens, the feeling of being overwhelmed can lead one to quit. Ruled by the all-or-nothing mentality, the thinking is that if the entire task cannot be completed then there is no point in doing any of it. This is a threat to your Spread-Workouts that you must be aware of.

If it looks like you are not going to get through all the reps you planned to do in a day, that's fine. Remind yourself that every rep counts and then *shrink* the task. If you have two hundred reps left to do for the day, do ten or twenty right away and then continue with what you were busy with. If you see another gap, do five or ten more. Breaking it down into very small numbers is an effective way of keeping on and pushing through. The take-home message is clear: *some is better than none, so never settle for less than a little.*

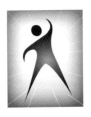

Endnotes

1. Chi Pang Wen and Xifeng Wu, Stressing Harms of Physical Inactivity to Promote Exercise, *The Lancet*, 18 July, 2012

2. Chi Pang Wen and Xifeng Wu, Stressing Harms of Physical Inactivity to Promote Exercise, *The Lancet*, 18 July, 2012

3. Woodcock J, Franco OH, Orsini N, Roberts I. Non-vigorous physical activity and all-cause mortality: systematic review and meta-analysis of cohort studies. *Int J Epidemiol* 2011; 40: 121–38.

4. Jakicic JM, Wing RR, Butler BA, Robertson RJ, Prescribing exercise in multiple short bouts versus one continuous bout: effects on adherence, cardiorespiratory fitness, and weight loss in overweight women. *International Journal of Obesity* 1995, (12):893-901

5. James A. Levine and Selene Yeager. *Move a Little, Lose a Lot* (New York: Three Rivers Press, 2009): 6.